KU-350-010

HOMOEOPATHY

An introduction to and explanation of Homoeopathy written especially for the layman and interested allopathic doctor. The author draws upon his thirty years of experience in practice to illustrate examples of the types of remedies used, the principles of taking the case and assessing the symptoms.

By the same author
ARNICA: THE AMAZING HEALER

HOMOEOPATHY
An Introductory Guide

by

A.C. Gordon Ross, M.B., Ch.B., M.F. Hom.

THORSONS PUBLISHERS LIMITED
Wellingborough, Northamptonshire

First published 1976
Eighth Impression 1986

© THORSONS PUBLISHERS LIMITED 1976

This book is sold subject to the condition that it shall not, by way of trade or otherwise, be lent, re-sold, hired out, or otherwise circulated without the publisher's prior consent in any form of binding or cover other than that in which it is published and without a similar condition including this condition being imposed on the subsequent purchaser.

ISBN 0 7225 0326 1

Printed in Great Britain by
Richard Clay (The Chaucer Press) Ltd,
Bungay, Suffolk

CONTENTS

Dedicated to the memory of my late partners, my brother Thomas Douglas Ross, M.B., Ch.B., F.F. Hom., and my brother-in-law, Thomas Landles Gordon, M.B., F.R.C.S., two fine prescribers who guided me into homoeopathy.

CHAPTER ONE

AN INTRODUCTION TO HOMOEOPATHY

The name comes from two Greek words *homois* – similar and *pathos* – suffering. Homoeopathy – spelt homeopathy in America – is a system of drug therapeutics elaborated by Dr Samuel Christian Hahnemann (1755-1843), who was born at Meissen in Germany. The principle of *similia similibus curentur* or 'like cures like' is a very old one and was noticed by Hippocrates, but it was left to Hahnemann to develop it with German tenacity, by testing more than a hundred remedies on himself.

His *Organon of the Art of Medicine* and his *Materia Medica Pura*, embodying his experiments with medicines on the human body (the first of their kind), are monuments of careful work, and with his massive *Chronic Diseases* are unique textbooks, if a little daunting in this age of no-leisure.

Hahnemann was a man of immense industry. After obtaining his Doctorate of Medicine, he made himself familiar with the new science of chemistry. The apothecaries of Leipzig rose up against him after he published his new method of medicine in 1796, when he denounced Polypharmacy – such things as Venetian treacle, with its innumerable ingredients. It was a threat to their business.

To swim against the tide of medical thought is an exhausting business, and Hahnemann was not an easy man to know. He was something of a recluse in Kothen, interested only in his ever-growing practice built solely on getting good results by individual treatment with single drugs. But as his fame grew he moved into the fashionable world of Paris, and gradually achieved international renown.

It is remarkable that this son of a poor china painter should have been able to attract wealthy, aristocratic patients from all the fashionable centres of Europe, and at the same time build up for himself an enormous practice among the poor in Paris, many of whom he treated free of charge. He was a classical scholar of no mean ability, a philologist, a botanist, and something of a dabler in Mesmerism in his later years. The best biography about him is the two-volume Samuel Hahnemann by Richard Haehl, MD, sometime physician to the Hahnemann Medical College of Philadelphia.

DEVELOPMENT IN BRITAIN

Hahnemann's system came to the attention of a Londoner, Dr Frederick Hervey Foster Quin, who became a convinced homoeopath, and was the first president of the British Homoeopathic Society from 1844 until his death in 1878. He once challenged the president of the Royal College of Physicians to a duel for slandering him – the president, however, declined the invitation.

The London Homoeopathic Hospital – now the Royal London Homoeopathic Hospital by virtue of Royal Patronage – was founded in 1850, four years before the great cholera epidemic reached London, having swept through Europe from Russia. The results of the treatment for that dread disease were so much better in the London Homoeopathic Hospital than elsewhere that some allopaths tried to have the statistics suppressed, though they were vouched for by the then minister of health.

Dr Quin had influential friends, however, and Lord Ebury published a separate Parliamentary Blue Book.

He was instrumental in protecting the right of homoeopathic doctors to practise their speciality, when the medical act of 1856 would have eliminated them altogether. Before that, students with homoeopathic leanings were refused their diplomas even though they had passed their examinations.

LONGER LIFE SPAN

Hahnemann died at the age of eighty-eight, which was in those days a remarkable age for a busy doctor to achieve. It has been pointed out to me by a correspondent in Canada that the average age at which homoeopathic doctors die is fully twenty years older than their allopathic colleagues, and this has been confirmed by the obituaries in *The British Medical Journal*.

In 1975 Dr Alva Benjamin, a distinguished London homoeopath, died at the age of ninety. The British Medical Journal for the same week showed the average age of death to be sixty-six.

Sir John Weir, K.C.V.O., G.C.V.O., M.B., Ch.B., died in April 1971 at the age of ninety-one. He was the doyen of the London homoeopaths, and was the personal physician to four monarchs, including the present Queen.

It seems more than a coincidence that this gentle, safe form of therapeutics, without side effects, should enable its practitioners to live well beyond their alloted span, as do most of their patients – a fact confirmed by the death certificates of homoeopathic doctors all over the world, for homoeopathy knows no frontiers. Britain, France, Germany, Italy, India, America, South America, Mexico, Russia, all have their followers of this form of treatment.

In Britain the Faculty of Homoeopathy was created by act of parliament in 1950 and homoeopathy was recognized as a speciality within the National Health Service, but whereas young doctors interested in other specialities are encouraged, and financed, by the National Health Service, the would-be homoeopath has to go it alone. Perhaps that is why there are less than 300 registered medical practitioners as fellows, members and associates of the faculty, but there is a wide following in the active British Homoeopathic Association, whose patrons include Sir Adrian Boult and Yehudi Menuhin.

'SCULPTING THE MIST'

In *Portrait of Europe* by Salvador De Madariaga, one-time Professor of Spanish Studies at Oxford, there is an admirable chapter, 'Germany and England', in which the author points out that for Germans, music is the supreme art, and that in Bach and Beethoven they attained form without matter, which is form at its aesthetic best. He says: 'Germans stand out as the particular nation with a philosophy dealing directly with the fluid nebulous atmosphere of thinking for the sake of thinking, and for the vigour and application they have devoted – to recall an admirable saying of Unamumo's – to the art of "Sculpting the Mist".'

Perhaps it is no accident, then, that Hahnemann was a German, that two of the world's most famous musicians are interested in homoeopathy, and that in another great country – India – there are many qualified homoeopathic doctors.

Mark the phrase, 'Sculpting the Mist'. Surely, as homoeopaths, that is what we have been doing for more than 200 years? We have practical experience, we know we get tangible results from a variety of our drugs – plants, minerals, spiders, metals, trees, herbs – which we attenuate to such an extent that for many years competent scientists have refused to believe that they have value. The infinitesimal dose is the stumbling block to the materially-minded, and will require a chapter to itself.

Hahnemann grew increasingly disenchanted with the state of medicine in the eighteenth century. When translating Cullen's *Materia Medica*, he started to ponder the use of Chinchona bark (*Quinine*) for the treatment of the ague, and experimented with small doses of the bark upon himself. To his surprise, he found he could bring on all the symptoms of trembling, fever and sickness, and from this he started to work out an entirely new – or rather, long-since forgotten – concept of drug therapy which he began to prove empirically on himself and his friends. Thus he began to 'Sculpt the Mist'. The infinitesimal dose was not part of his philosophy at the time, but practical experience and the careful keeping of records on each individual treated showed him the value of the single drug given in the smallest amount to stimulate a reaction.

Only a German could have done it: a methodical German, interested in all things, including music and mathematics and pin-pointing the practical application of form without matter.

NOT FAITH HEALING

Homoeopathy will not die out, as many allopaths have hoped. One can fool some of the people all of the time and all of the people some of the time, but no one can fool all of the people all of the time: homoeopathy has existed for nearly 200 years, and every year more and more patients are grateful for the results obtained. It has been suggested, time after time, that homoeopathy is a kind of faith healing, but this is a very superficial judgement because it acts well on children – indeed, we often get our most dramatic results with young children, for their systems are not clogged up with a variety of medicaments, as is the case with the chronic sick.

Some of the results with animals are also truly astonishing, and animals can have little faith in the prescriber or his medicines. About ten years ago, an epidemic of gastro-enteritis ran through a chinchilla farm at Kilmalcolm in Renfrewshire, and two veterinary surgeons thought all the stock would have to be destroyed. In desperation, the owner phoned me and she was sent a packet of *Arsenicum album* in low potency to put in the drinking water, for the little beasts had a great thirst. A few of the worst affected died, but three-quarters of her valuable stock was saved.

The *Scottish Sunday Express* of 17 December 1967 reported on the serious foot-and-mouth epidemic running through Cheshire and Shropshire, when about 100 farmers acted on my suggestion and gave *Borax* (sodium tetra hydrate) as a prophylactic to their cattle, so that in dairy farms many cows escaped being slaughtered. *Borax* did not act so well in mixed farms, where the preventative was not so easily administered.

These are just two incidents in a lifetime of homoeopathic practice, which illustrate the fact that homoeopathy is more than faith healing.

The late Raymond Mortimer once wrote: 'The venom with which succeeding historians have treated Macaulay is easily comprehensible. He committed the sin that to professional men is unforgivable, he opened the arcana to the general public.' Perhaps that is why our great profession loves medical jargon, and does little to encourage books like this one, written solely to give thoughtful people some idea of another approach to health.

CHAPTER TWO

HOMOEOPATHY COMPARED WITH ALLOPATHY

It was suggested that this chapter should be headed 'Homoeopathy versus Allopathy', but I dislike the word 'versus' – it smacks too much of competition or a football match. After all, any doctor worth his salt has entered what has been described as 'the most distinterested profession in the world', with an earnest desire to help suffering humanity. He is subjected to a long period of training – some of it quite useless, in my opinion – and if his professors ever mention the word homoeopathy, they do so in a derogatory fashion and label it Quackery.

That is why homoeopaths tend to run in families, and only if students have actual experience of its benefits can they be persuaded to study the system. Most of them are so exhausted by getting their degrees that they are daunted by our old-fashioned textbooks, they hesitate to enter a second long course of study, and the clever ones tend to go in for the various specialities as the first step towards a consultant post.

With this in mind, let us examine Hahnemann's four ideas, which I think are sound and still applicable to modern medicine. An idea should be thought of as a mental image. This is the proper meaning of the word, as defined by the great Dr Samuel Johnson in his dictionary.

Hahnemann's first idea, or mental image, is to think of the patient as an individual, a trilogy of body, mind and spirit, and that treatment must be directed to help all three facets of personality, with his own peculiar reactions.

His second idea is to regard disease as dis-ease or disharmony, meaning a state of disorder in the person, and not a label to attach to symptoms, signs and clinical findings.

His third idea is to think of drugs as restorers of harmony, and not as lethal weapons to destroy the bacilli and cocci, which nature surely put into the world for a better purpose than to be destroyed by man's ingenuity.

Finally, his fourth mental image is to realize that the body can maintain its own defence against lethal weapons in the shape of heavy drugging, and that the patient's Vital Force can often withstand infection by its mechanisms, such as fever, which will burn out the infection if left alone.

FOUR IMAGES COMPARED WITH ALLOPATHIC APPROACH

Let us now elaborate on these four ideas about treatment in some detail and, where possible, compare them with the allopathic approach to disease.

We must not only accept the mental image of the patient as a whole person, but must also think of him as an individual; everyone is different, with personalities, palates, prejudices and peccadilloes. The person best qualified to treat a patient is the doctor who knows most about him. He must know something about his family, his heredity, his environment, his previous illnesses, his financial worries. Such knowledge is not usually available to the consultant to whom he is referred, who may know nothing of the patient's circumstances, who gets no help from the panel doctor's polite little note, but who knows everything about say slipped discs – perhaps the only symptom presented to the consultant.

The second idea – to regard dis-ease as disharmony

– means that we must accept the fact that it is not the actual bacteria which makes the patient ill, but the weight of attack of the invaders. This is a hard idea for allopaths to grasp. In other words, organisms may live in a state of symbiosis in the body, and it is only when the balance is disturbed or the Vital Force weakened that one crop of bacteria multiply at the expense of another, so endangering the life of the patient. It is when the experienced homoeopath encounters this state of affairs that he uses the modern weapons of the allopath, the antibiotics – the sulpha drugs, the cortizone derivatives and so on.

But we believe that if these drugs are used without discrimination, viruses become more virulent and weird side effects take place, thus prolonging the illness unnecessarily. In my last years in practice I came across a peculiarly virulent type of virus pneumonia which was never encountered in the pre-penicillin days.

The third mental image is getting into the habit of regarding all drugs as harmony restorers and not as lethal weapons. The good homoeopath rarely makes the body into a desert and calls it peace – by killing off the bowel microbes with tetracycline in an illness such as gastro-enteritis, for instance. He uses as few drugs as possible and rarely mixes them, and he never interferes with improvement in the patient's condition, but lets the Vital Force take over. If we accept our first three mental images, we can accept our fourth, which is that bacteria breed their own immunity to the various chemical agents used to kill them. At first it was thought that venereal disease could be wiped out entirely by penicillin. The chemists made more and more efficient types of penicillin and yet we hear that V.D. is on the increase again, and that penicillin has little or no effect on the gonococcus now.

In my opinion, what is wrong with allopathic medicine today is that its adherents have never sat down and developed a philosophy of healing. Hippocrates was the true father of the idea that 'like cures like'. Orthodox medicine took the wrong turning some 500 years later, when it elected to follow others who developed the idea that all disease should be fought by antidotes, and had no thought for the Vital Force or the harmony that exists in the human body. Perhaps they are to blame for the flood of medicaments which daily go down the throats of the great unsuspecting public, to the delight of the great pharmaceutical chemists and the despair of those accountants in the National Health Service.

IMPRESSIVE ADVANCES
Surely there is a better way of coping with illness than by giving an infinite amount of medicine, often for trivial illness? Homoeopaths, however, must not be churlish about the impressive advanced made by the orthodox schools of medicine in the last decades. Tuberculosis has almost been wiped out, as has diphtheria and scarlet fever, and the treatment of mental illness has advanced enormously since the last war. Yet there remain great areas of illness where the allopath can only palliate the patient. Enteritis, allergies, skin diseases, rheumatism in all its varieties, bronchitis, catarrhs, influenzas, the common cold, shingles, are but a few of the common ailments which respond to homoeopathy much more quickly and permanently than to orthodox treatment.

The great American literary figure, Oliver Wendell Holmes, passed a very superficial judgement on homoeopathy when he said that, as far as he could judge, all the good in the new system was due to stopping the mixed strong medicine in vogue in his generation. Another reproach often levelled against it by orthodox physicians is that we have made no contributions to medical knowledge since the time of Hahnemann. That is hardly accurate.

It was in fact our own Dr Dudgeon who invented the Sphygmomanometer, that invaluable instrument for testing the blood pressure; Professor J.T. Kent, M.A., M.D., (attached in his lifetime to at least six homoeopathic teaching hospitals in America) who developed the first true philosophy of healing and tried out and tested many new drugs; and the late Dr W.E. Boyd of Glasgow whose important researches into electrical phenomena convinced many of the actuality of the minimum dose.

Dr Bach and Dr John Paterson both put into their lifetimes some great work on the non-lactose fermenting organisms of the bowel. Some observers have said this work is of infinite value in the early study of chronic disease, for their nosodes and bowel-culture remedies altered the soil on which disease grew. Homoeopaths have also shown a better way to practical application of herbal remedies by a close study of the ancient herbal lore, and have taken the good medical properties of trees, plants, flowers and weeds and, by potentization, used them for the good of mankind.

DETAILED INDIVIDUAL TREATMENT

Perhaps, however, our main usefulness rests in the careful application, at the bedside and in the consulting room, of principles laid down 200 years ago by Samuel Hahnemann. He always stressed the importance of the individual, of taking long and careful notes about every aspect of his character and illness, and of the effect of the single remedy on his condition.

With a large panel list, individual treatment is not easy. The overworked doctor cannot take adequate notes on his patients, whom he rarely knows personally, and if a case is dealt with by assistants the patient feels lost. If by any chance anything seriously wrong is suspected, or if a boil or carbuncle has to be opened or a finger lanced, the patient is at once referred to the nearest hospital. The juniors in a practice are terrified of being sued, so will not take responsibility.

Patients with chronic stomach trouble, diagnosed in hospital as an ulcer, have to wait weeks for the result of their X-rays and sometimes years before they get a postcard to go for their operation. It is no one's fault; it is the result of bureaucratic control. But one of Hahnemann's fundamental principles has been lost – the patient feels diminished as an individual.

Contrast this with the worried accountant or tax collector who goes to a homoeopathic physician because he is suffering from pains in his stomach, an excessive amount of flatulence, and sits down to his meals feeling very hungry but is quickly satisfied with a few bites of food. He looks prematurely aged with furrowed brow and sunken lines on his face, and his hair has turned grey years ago. The pains are worse on the right side and are always worse in the evening. Ninety-nine out of a hundred Homoeopaths would give him *Lycopodium* (club moss), and be certain that they could help him – his pains, his tiredness, his perpetual worried state of mind. The dominant school say the *Lycopodium* spores are quite inert. They have never taken the trouble to crush the spores and experiment with them in minute doses.

It has been said that homoeopaths are mere symptom coverers – that they do not bother about diagnosis. This is not so – the good homoeopath gets to know the face of disease as in the above example. Even if the patient has a peptic ulcer, surely it is worth while for the doctor to try him on *Lycopodium*, which to his certain knowledge has helped many similar patients before? The experienced homoeopath has learned what his medicines are capable of, he has got to know his drugs as a father knows his children, and if occasionally he is disappointed, it is not the drug that is to blame but the fact that he has not matched the drug perfectly to the symptoms.

He will then retake the case and perhaps find out that the patient's wife has been given a present of a set of aluminium pots and pans, which she uses with enthusiasm. It so happens that a very few of the population are susceptible to the oxide of aluminium, which gives them heartburn and no desire to eat, and the doctor's unpopular advice is to revert to the old-fashioned enamel. This is the kind of thing that makes the young housewife say the doctor is a crank – but he is only talking from experience.

ANIMAL PRODUCTS

Homoeopathic medicines have been proved or tested time and time again on healthy persons, which means there has seldom been occasion to subject animals to experiment. We do, however, use animal products in our medicines. A good example of this is *Latrodectus mactans*, the black-widow spider, so called because it kills its partner after mating. It lurks about outside privies in warm countries and often bites victims in their private parts. In a few minutes the unfortunate becomes shocked, giving an almost textbook picture of angina pectoris, with violent pain down the left arm, laboured breathing, ashy colour and every appearance that the end is near. Thus we use it for angina, often with good effect if given soon enough.

We also use snake venoms such as *Lachesis* (The Bushmaster of Surucucu) which is a good remedy for delirium tremens, where there is much trembling and confusion. Strangely enough, it is much used by us for the chatty type of elderly female who comes to us with bruised blood under the skin. *Lachesis* decomposes the blood and causes haemorrhages.

Another of the common female remedies, quite unknown to the orthodox school, is *Sepia* – the brown juice of the cuttle fish. This acts chiefly on the portal system, but has many curious mental symptoms.

There are a few animal products which by potentization, become active for suffering humanity – indeed, homoeopathy can make preparations from practically any substance, including minerals like gold, copper, zinc, lead and platinum.

WIDELY-USED REMEDIES

Some of the most widely-used homoeopathic medicines are: *Aconite* for sudden chills; *Arnica* for bruises; *Arsenicum alb.* for gastro-enteritis; *Bryonia* for rheumatic pains the worse for movement; *Rhus toxicodendron* for rheumatic pains the worse for rest; *Nux vomica* for stomach upsets; *Sulphur* for skin complaints; *Gelsemium* for influenzas. Many missionaries going to remote parts take a small case of such medicines with them and learn to use them well. They get to know the scope of the medicines and, provided they use them in low potencies, if they do no good, they can do no harm. Potencies will be dealt with in a later chapter – they are a stumbling block to the materially-minded scientist, though less so now than in the past.

Homoeopaths are sometimes accused of being secretive in their choice of remedies, because when someone receiving, say, instant relief from a blinding headache, tells a neighbour and that neighbour phones the doctor and asks for the medicine that helped Mrs Brown, he has to say that he cannot merely prescribe the same thing for her. As has been stressed, homoeopathy is individual treatment and what helped Mrs Smith may have no effect on Mrs Brown, who will require to have her case taken thoroughly and all symptoms noted.

How does a homoeopath cope with the symptoms in a new patient? It is perhaps best to start with food – this makes the patient less nervous, and is a subject of universal interest. For instance, does the patient know of any food which aggravates his trouble, such as milk, eggs, onions, or shell-fish?

Incidentally, long ago I had a consultation with a nervous little man accompanied by his large aggressive wife. Asked what meat he ate most of, he thought for a minute and replied 'Mince'. Did that give him stomach pains? At once his formidable wife broke in: 'He only gets mince about once a week doctor, and that's because its cheaper than steaks.' He had taken many anti-acid tablets and for his first visit got *Nux vomica*, which helped to clear the picture for his constitutional remedy, which was *Argentum nitricum*. He had been x-rayed four times and no ulcer had been found, but he would eventually have gone to ulceration, for worry, hurry and curry was his background, plus a wife who domineered. He got relief by drinking cold water.

I asked about condiments and whether he liked fat (a craving for fat is a useful pointer in suspected gall-bladder cases). I went down from mouth to anus, questioning all the way, and eventually went from what we call the particulars to the generals – those that the patient feels is his very being. Was he chilly; afraid; worse at certain times of the day? The little man said on his first visit that his stomach was always worse in the winter. Aggravation by cold is a *Nux* symptom, but it is not always a reliable one, for on his second visit he said a hot summer upset him more than a cold winter, and that is covered by *Argentum nit.*

HOT AND COLD REMEDIES

From the foregoing it can be seen that the doctor must know his drugs thoroughly. Almost the first things I had to learn by heart were the hot and cold remedies. There are many more remedies predominantly aggravated by cold than by hot, of which the common ones are the *Calciums* and *Arsenicum, Causticum, Phosphorus* and *Rhus tox.*

The art of prescribing – and it is an art more than a science – is spotting the patients that run to type. It takes a lot of patience and cannot be done in a hurry – it takes about an hour to get all the particulars and generals out of a new patient. Sometimes the doctor feels it is like looking for a needle in a haystack but patient spade-work is rarely without clues.

The important remedies aggravated by heat are *Argentum nit., Natrum mur., Pulsatilla,* and *Sulphur.* The *Natrum mur.* types are the worst to spot on a first interview. They are usually joyless women with a negative attitude to life, and this is a symptom in itself. *Natrum muriaticum,* which is nothing but common salt, is one of the best remedies for a certain type of female headache – the blinding type that lasts all day.

TREATING THE COMMON COLD

Writing of *Natrum mur.* brings the common cold to mind. It is surprising how lightly our profession regards this ailment and yet it is often the initial cause of much ill health and loss of time at work. Colds should not be suppressed except by homoeopathic remedies. One old practitioner once said to me, 'I tell my patients that it will take three days to incubate, three days to endure it, and three days for it to go away.' Certainly, it is better to have this philosophy than to give aspirin or penicillin to reduce the temperature, for the temperature is nature's way of burning infection out of the body.

Colds can be caused by infection, emotion, chills, over-tiredness or worry, or the patient having a tendency to catch cold due to chronic catarrh. Other causes are dampness in an unfavourable environment, or wearing the wrong clothes – most people wear too many clothes.

Homoeopaths have at least a dozen remedies which have a great reputation for cutting short the common cold. *Aconite* is the best remedy at the start of a cold in the *Aconite* type of person, who is usually plethoric and over-anxious, and has probably come down with a chill waiting for transport in a cold east wind. *Allium cepa* is good for the sudden streamer with acrid discharge from the nose.

Arsenicum alb. helps those thin, watery discharges which excoriate the upper lip, and colds where the nose is stuffed and not relieved by sneezing. *Natrum mur.* is used for the emotional type of cold with much watery sneezing. I had a patient who got a cold of this type every time she had a row with her husband. *Dulcamara* alleviates those colds occurring in the cold, wet weather of early winter, accompanied by rheumatism and sore red eyes. *Gelsemium* is prescribed almost automatically when the patient phones up and says he feels he is in for a dose of flu, aching in every bone. *Nux vomica* is for a dry-weather type of cold when the patient is irritable, chilly, and full of flatulence and resentment.

Phosphorus is useful for the stopping-and-starting

type of cold in the tall, sensitive, red-haired person who usually has poor resistance to streptococci, has a history of tonsillitis, scarlet fever and many nose bleeds, and who is narrow-chested. *Hepar sulph.* is a good remedy for the type of patient who starts sneezing in cold winds. Here the discharge starts watery but soon thickens up. *Kali bich.* is a suitable remedy when the discharge becomes ropy and tough, and comes out in long strings. *Pulsatilla* and *Sepia* are both good catarrhal remedies but only for the typical persons suitable for them.

Bacillinum is an excellent nosode for clearing up the remains of a lingering catarrh, while *Cistus canadensis* is a good (but neglected) remedy for post-nasal catarrh (catarrh between the nose and throat), especially if the patient has a craving for cheese.

Most of these remedies are easy to study, and if the prescriber gets a good idea of the type of patient on whom they act best, he should do good work with potency 30 in any of them. If the patient is desperately cold and cannot get warm, a dose of *Camphor 30* may abort a chill, and if such a chill is due to an unexpected ducking in cold water, *Bellis* should be considered.

Patients who will not react to any of these cold remedies are the chronic catarrhal types who have had their septa straightened, their tonsils and adenoids removed, and every available bit of mucosal nose lining removed by surgery. If these unfortunates pick up a virulent infection, the early defences of the body are no longer there to cope with it and the trouble goes further.

The hay fever type of cold looks simple but it is difficult to treat for it is an allergy which can be activated by pollen, by animals, by sunlight, or by temperature. I give hay fever patients a prophylactic dose of Timothy grass early in the season and in early June, and employ the intervening time looking for their constitutional remedy. In women, it is surprising how often that remedy is *Natrum mur*. Men, on the other hand, are often of the psoric type requiring *Sulphur, Calc. carb.* and *Lycopodium* in that order.

Dr W. Ritchie McCrae had this to say about the common cold:

> A very interesting fact keeps recurring in the practice of Homoeopathy. We refer to the common cold. It is not claimed that Homoeopathy holds the secret of cure for the common cold. It would appear that the cold is an exhibition of the commonly held good resistance of a healthy individual and when such a person goes through the routine of eliminating such an infection, he does so with little or no disturbance to his general health, and is quite capable of carrying on his normal life. The interesting point is that patients report, quite often, that they have received treatment from potentized medicines for ordinary everyday complaints, not necessarily for respiratory troubles at all, and they find that to their pleasure and astonishment they no longer suffer from their usual periodic disabling colds.
>
> This may seem to be a minor detail in the practice of medicine but it also comes forward to show the far-reaching constitutional influence of good therapy. It is a foundation stone to the edifice of preventative medicine. If potentized medicines achieve this success in what might seem to be minor detail, why should we not consider its benefit to be endowed upon many, if not all, other aspects of disease?
>
> (*British Homoeopathic Journal*, July 1961)

We cannot leave the common cold without saying something about coughs. We all have our favourite medicines for coughs, which seem more common today than ever before. I remember an old practitioner who once said: 'Think of six medicines for dry coughs; *Aconite, Belladonna, Bryonia, Nux vomica, Phosphorus, Rumex*; and for loose, wet coughs: *Pulsatilla, Sepia,*

Stannum, Calcarea, Kali carbonicum, and *Kali bichronicum.'*

This is nice, neat division to impress students looking for short cuts but it is not good homoeopathic teaching, in which one should never prescribe on a single symptom, but on the totality. For instance, I can remember a patient who was red-eyed and sneezy with a hoarse voice and the kind of cough that brought up little phlegm with great effort. He got *Senega* (snakewort),' not one of our great cough medicines, but one which gave him great ease within a day.

THE FOUR-LEGGED STOOL

When teaching homoeopathy, my own mentor, tried to get a firm base for the prescription – a kind of four-legged stool. This is what is meant by the totality of symptoms. In the case mentioned above, *Senega,* was chosen because of the hoarse voice, the red eyes, the cough that always ended in a sneeze, and the difficulty the old chap had in getting anything up. But no one can possibly remember all the symptoms attached to a remedy and this is where the repertories are invaluable. The best is Dr Kent's repertory, but the handy one is Boericke's. A repertory is a storehouse, or index, of symptoms. One should never be ashamed of using it in the presence of the patient, for the human memory cannot carry all the symptoms, or the drugs related thereto.

I can recollect an old lady telling her sister: 'Your doctor cannot be much good – he has to refer to a book before he decides on what medicine to give you!' I deflated the interfering one with two aphorisms: 'Ability is the power of applying knowledge to practical purposes, and all improvements in memory come from better methods of recording facts!'

Kent's repertory runs to 1,422 pages and records innumerable symptoms and related drugs. This is an area where the computer could perhaps be of service, by making dispensary work much easier, when many patients have to be seen in a morning, real homoeopathy – the treatment of the individual case – gets little chance to succeed; though it is surprising how the experienced homoeopath, by knowing what his drugs are capable of doing and by recognizing the face of disease, can often come up with a helpful remedy in a few minutes.

Lord Cohen of Birkenhead once wrote in *The Sunday Times*:

The two dominant and inter-related trends in the medicine of the 19th and 20th centuries have been increasing specialization and the application of the instruments of the basic sciences, Physics, Chemistry, and Biology, to the investigation of disease. This has led over a wide field to an impersonalization of medicine in which there has been the risk of the disease being regarded as more important than the patient.

Not so in homoeopathy, where the patient has always been thought of as more important than his disease or disharmony. People are more important than things.

CHAPTER THREE

POTENCY AND THE MINIMUM DOSE

Both these homoeopathic conceptions are difficult to explain and difficult for the layman to understand.

Towards the end of the eighteenth century, Hahnemann started treatment with what might be called material doses which could be measured, such as one-tenth of a gramme of arsenic in treating involuntary diarrhoeas, but ten years later he worked with much smaller doses, simply because he found he got better results. His ever diminishing doses brought upon him the wrath of the powerful apothecaries and the ridicule of those engaged in the new science of inorganic chemistry, and thus did much to damage homoeopathy for the next hundred years.

We should get clear in our minds that the idea of the actual principle of homoeopathy, *similia similibus curentur*, does not depend on either potency theory, or on the minimum dose. We are practising a kind of crude homoeopathy when we rub a frostbitten foot with snow, or when we eat an onion to ward off a head cold, or when, the morning after we have dined not wisely but too well, we take a prairie-oyster to get things going again. 'The hair of the dog' is the popular name for this kind of treatment.

It is important to have a clear idea what homoeopaths mean by the use of the word 'potency'. It is the latent power of a medicine developed, or made available, by repeated dilutions and by trituration or succussion.

Trituration is the act of reducing a substance to a fine powder by rubbing, bruising, pounding or crushing: galvanizing is perhaps a better word, more in line with the idea of releasing hidden energy. *Lycopodium* (club moss), for example, is made active by crushing the spores, and the pestle and mortar have been used by medical men since the seventeenth century, for pounding substances to a fine powder. They stand now as a symbol of their trade on many consulting-room mantlepieces. Succussion is the act of continual shaking – not stirring – to distribute the particles of a substance evenly throughout a solution.

THE DEGREE OF DILUTION
One of Glasgow's most distinguished consultants once

said to me: 'They tell me you chaps believe that if you put a pinch of common salt into the Clyde at Glasgow Bridge, you can take it out at Greenock and expect it to cure a headache.' This is the kind of ridicule that was hard to take in the old days.

The late Dr William Boyd of Glasgow proved that mercuric chloride had potency when diluted to such an extent that there was no trace of the molecule left, and his methods for investigating the action of micro-doses of mercuric chloride on the hydrolysis of soluble starch with malt diastase were fully reported in homoeopathic literature in the years just after the second World War. I had the privilege of living next door to Dr Boyd for twenty years, and can recollect watching him demonstrate on his electronic biological heart rate recorder how a frog's heart would respond to the drug *Strophantus hispidus* (kombe seed) in a minute homoeopathic dose – and yet *Strophantus* is regarded as a muscle poison.

In the *Daily Telegraph* of 19 August 1954, under the heading: 'Research Reveals New Force in Physics', there is a report of some of Dr Boyd's work. One paragraph reads: 'The power of the solution does not depend solely on the degree of dilution, but on a special progressive method in its preparation, the energy latent in the drug is apparently liberated and increased by a forceful shaking of the liquid at each stage of the process.'

It is not the purpose in this book to go into the mysteries of potentization. Reams have been written about it both here and in America, where a new discipline has arisen – the Pharmacology of the Infinitesimal. Dr Pulford of Toledo, U.S.A., has stated: 'The more one studies the mystery of potentization, the more one is forced to the belief that the chemical action, as related to the drug, concerns the material physical confines of the drug proper, only, and not the drug proper itself. This is forced on to us by the fact that as the drug is potentized – as the container recedes from the bulk state, the chemical reaction becomes less pronounced. Yet in ratio, as the visible container or base disappears, the dynamic or curative power of the drug, properly increases.' Then in another place, in the same paper, he states: 'Then all our potentization does to the drug proper in any way, is to reduce its physical restrainer to a point where the real drug is the more readily freeable and accessible.'

This seems to me to be a fair assessment and brings us into the realm of the permeability of cell membranes, and to the thought that potentization, which Hahnemann found out by accident, is a means of separating the structural informational content of a chemical from its associated chemical mass. As Dr G.O. Barnard states, 'Hahnemann, with his particular method of dilution with succussion, quite fortuitously exposed a natural phenomenon of profound biological significance.'

CALCULATING THE POTENCY

Potencies are calculated on the decimal or, more commonly, the centesimal scale, and they rise by geometrical progression. In the decimal series, one part of the drug in nine parts of distilled water and alcohol – is shaken up (by mechanical means these days) and this gives a strength of one in ten, or 1x. One drop of this solution is added to nine parts of the solvent and succussed to give 2x, and the process is repeated to give 3x, which is known as a low potency. The procedure can be continued *ad infinitum* to give what are called the high potencies. Similarly, for the centesimal series, one drop of the mother tincture – say, *Arnica* – is added to ninety-nine drops of the solvent and succussed many times to give 1c; the process is repeated with one drop of resultant solution to give 2c, and so on. 2x and 1c both represent one part in a hundred.

It has been established by the mathematicians that at about the tenth centesimal dilution, there will be no molecules left of the original substance, but homoeopaths believe the energy is still there. We do not yet understand the philosophy behind the theory of the infinitely small.

Professor William Burridge, M.A., M.D., wrote upon this matter as a distinguished physiologist. In one paper he quoted Dr Zaidi, who experimented with nicotinic acid. He found the acid active up to a dilution of one part in one thousand millions. As Professor Burridge says, 'A dilution of 10^{12} or one part in a billion is very small: it represents adding a quart of fluid to a lake five miles long, one mile broad and some 300 feet deep, yet in such great dilutions some drugs may act.'

This materialist outlook was the one held by the Glasgow consultant when he made his sarcastic remark, but he was too old to appreciate thermo-dynamics, the phenomenon of radiation, and while he may have known molecules were made up of atoms, he did not know atoms could be split into protons and electrons to release an energy which saved the world from disaster in the Second World War.

The minimum dose is the lowest potency that can provoke a reaction in the patient and this is often a matter of professional preference on the part of the practitioner. A safe rule for the beginner is to use low potencies (which can be repeated often) for acute work, and keep the high potencies for chronic cases where the constitutional remedy is known by familiarity with all the patient's circumstances.

From about 1793 to 1828, Hahnemann worked with mother tinctures and low potencies such as 3x, and some experienced practitioners such as Dr Duncan Cameron of Bristol, accustomed in his busy practice to use high potencies 30c-200c-1m (1m is one part in 10^{-2000}) ran a most interesting experiment in the early 'fifties where he and his partners used low potencies with good results. Low potencies were within the understanding of the experimenters with homoeopathic medicines, and it was only with experience that they realized the tremendous potential, or energy, in dilutions.

CHAPTER FOUR

THE VITAL FORCE AND CHRONIC DISEASE

On the subject of the Hunza tribe in the valley of the Himalayan Mountains, who are reputed to live to an average of 130 years without the aid of doctors or chemists, Dr Bernard writes: 'They drink from birth, untouched water full of sludge that has splashed down mountain rocks over many kinds of vegetation. Are we witnessing in fact, a natural situation in which an extremely large number of remedies are being potentized to provide the waters of life?' (G.O. Barnard, D.Sc., Ph.D., M.I.E.E., *Journal of the American Institute of Homoeopathy*, Vol. 58, Nos. 7 and 8, 1965.) This is an interesting concept, but hardly in line with the Hahnemannian dictum of the single remedy, never repeated while improvements last.

But in my opinion, the Hunzas are endowed with what Hahnemann meant by the Vital Force; a quality which modern medicine unwittingly suppresses by over-medication of its patients. It has been said that a quarter of admissions to our hospitals today result from iatrogenic illness – that is, illness produced by the doctor, or the patient himself, from over-medication. It is too easy for patients to persuade the doctor to hand out prescriptions for every new panacea that comes on to the market, with the result that his system becomes clogged with medicines.

When I was young, it was only laxatives. Almost every elderly patient was conditioned, by specious advertising, to think that constipation was something to avoid at all costs, with the result that many took a laxative every night of their lives. They then got 'hooked' on them and the bowels refused to work naturally.

That was one benefit of being brought up in a homoeopathic household. In our medicine cabinet there were only a few bottles: tincture of *Arnica*, for bruises (Mrs Beeton's favourite); tincture of *Calendula*, for cuts; tincture of *Urtica*, for burns; tincture of *Ledum*, for stings; *Nux vomica* 6c, for stomach upsets; *Arsenicum album* 6c, for diarrhoeas; *Aconite* 6c, for early colds; *Gelsemium* 6c, for influenzas. We became familiar with them and rarely required anything else. Sleeping pills, pep pills, tranquillizers, pills to reduce weight, pills for headaches, were quite unknown to us, and we were the better for it.

HAHNEMANN'S 'LIFE FORCE'

Hahnemann put most of his early thoughts into his *Organon*. Classical scholars will recognize this word as the title of Aristotle's *Instrument of All Reasoning* – J.M. Dent and Sons, published the *Organon* in Everyman's Library and it can still be picked up in second-hand bookshops.) In paragraph 227 we find that he assumes the existence of a Life Force, which is liberated by the homoeopathic remedy. Bergson called it the 'Elan

Vital', and Smuts called it 'Holism'.

Dr Ledermann has pointed out that the vitalistic
view is shared by the school of natural therapy, which
uses unspecific forms of treatment, such as dieting,
hydrotherapy and heliotherapy. – (E.K. Ledermann,
M.D., F.F.Hom., 'Body, Mind and Spirit', *British
Homoeopathic Journal*, October 1961.)

In Paragraph 13 in the *Organon*, occurs this passage:

All that mankind has apprehended of animal magnetism,
galvanism, electricity, attraction and repulsion, earth
magnetism, caloric, phenomena of gases, and other objects of
chemical and physical enquiry, is far, far wide of the
comprehensive, clear and fruitful explanation of even the
smallest function of the living organism, whether healthy or
diseased. What innumerable, unknown powers and their laws
may be involved in the regulation of the living organs, powers
and laws, of which we know nothing and for whose recognition
we should need infinitely more and infinitely finer senses than
we have.

In his article, Dr Ledermann goes on to point out:

Hahnemann did affirm that the body works as a whole. He
said: 'The human body is, in its living state, a unity, a complete
and rounded whole. Every sensation, every manifestation of
force, every inter-relation of the material of one part is
intimately concerned with the sensation, force manifestations
and inter-relations of all the other parts; no part can suffer
without involving all the rest in suffering (greater or less) and in
alteration.'

From this holistic conception follows Hahnemann's
insistence that a patient's habits of life must be regulated and
'all harmful influences and errors in the mode of life' should be
eliminated. These principles are in line with Natural Therapy.

If we accept the idea of wholeness for the purpose of
understanding life, without making it into an entity, without
presupposing a holistic force, we avoid the standpoint of
vitalistic metaphysics. We then follow Kant who considered
purposiveness and teleology not as a constitutive but as a
regulative principle which guides our understanding of living
organisms.

I accept the Kantian point of view, as it avoids dogmatism which is characteristic of both the materialistic and vitalistic metaphysical points of view.

THE HISTORY OF THE IDEA

Today modern medicine has divorced itself from philosophy and we must go back a long way in history to find the reason and the thought process which enabled science to take control of the art of medicine.

The idea of that elusive thing – the Vital Force – was known to Hippocrates, born on the island of Cos in 460 B.C. He was known as the father of medicine, responsible for eighty-seven philosophic papers, and for his Hippocratic Oath, which used to be taken by all medical students.

Claudius Galenus, born at Pergamum, Mysia, in A.D. 130 was the greatest authority on medicine for the next 500 years. He supported Hippocrates and his ideas, and at Cambridge University in the fourteenth century, it was compulsory for medical students to attend two courses of lectures on Galen's *Commentaries on Hippocrates* and his writing.

With the coming of the barbarians to western Europe in the fifth and sixth centuries, however, Galen's teaching died out. The conquering Arabs acquired some of his ideas and after their Spanish conquests, the Arabic version of Galen's *Commentaries* came back to mediaeval Europe, but in Latin translations all mixed up with Eastern lore, herbal lore, and smatterings of the occult sciences.

After the Norman Conquest in 1066, this influence of Arabian teaching reached England. Until well on in the sixteenth century all English medical theory was based on faulty Arabic versions of Plato, Aristotle, Empedocles, Galen, and Hippocrates, with a fair sprinkling of Arabic magic and astrology, and traces of Hindu philosophy and Chinese medical lore. For example, Chaucer, in his description of the Doctor of Physics, records how the twelve signs of the zodiac are related to the various parts of the body. (*Prologue*, 413-36).

Medicine's link with astronomy can be traced back to Empedocles who tried to postulate that the constitution of the human body was part of the general question of the constitution of matter. He was the first to suggest the four elements, Air, Earth, Fire, and Water. Aristotle added a fifth, later to be called by the Latin word 'quintessence', of which the stars and the souls of men were composed. Shakespeare, who read much medical lore made Cleopatra say, just before she committed suicide:

> I am fire and air, my other elements
> I give to baser life.

The Ancients thought that the perfect man was one in whom the elements were mixed in perfect proportion. In *Julius Caesar*, Shakespeare made Antony say of Brutus:

> His life was gentle, and the elements
> So mixed in him, that nature might stand up
> And say to all the world, 'This was a Man!'

Here we see the first evidence that health was harmony – and that there was a Vital Force in nature combining the elements. Shakespeare thought that putrefaction of humours resulted in imposthumes (abscesses), as we see in *Hamlet*:

> This is the imposthume of much wealth and peace
> That inwards breaks, and shows no cause without
> Why the man dies.

Pope, too, knew the importance of the mind and environment on the health:

> Imagination plies her dangerous art
> And pours it all upon the peccant part.

I often think of this couplet when trying to convince a women she has not got cancer of the breast.

THE MOST IMPORTANT NUTRIMENT

Hippocrates said that the body is sustained and supported by three kinds of nutriment, food, drink and spirit, of which the last is by far the most important. An example in our own time is Sir Francis Chichester who was said to have cancer, yet his spirit supported him through a long, lone sail around the world. If this was not the Vital Force, I know of no other name to call it.

Democritus (430 B.C.) thought that the various attributes of the soul were located in particular organs in the body – thought in the brain, anger in the heart, desire in the liver, and laughter in the spleen. The materialistic scientists had little use for this ancient history. Once Leewenhoek of Delft had invented the microscope and microbes could be seen, science was convinced that they were on firm ground, and disease could be eradicated by killing off invaders.

Many years ago I attended a fine old lady who had a young Highland lass as her maid. This girl was twenty-six, tall, dark and strong, and a great help to her mistress, until one day she suddenly took to her bed. I was asked to see her and could find nothing wrong. She was given *Natrum muriaticum*, for she seemed depressed. After two weeks she was no better so she was sent into hospital in Glasgow under one of our most brilliant physicians, where she had every test known to medical science. Everything was normal, but one day she turned her face to the wall and died.

It was a mystery until the old lady found among the

dead girl's possessions a letter from a policeman saying he could no longer take her out as he was a married man. She was the only genuine instance in my experience of someone dying of a broken heart – the will to live had gone.

If she had confessed her trouble she would have been given *Ignatia* (St Ignatius Bean), which has a reputation for helping long-lasting grief, but she was uncooperative and would not tell me a single symptom.

THREE GROUPS OF CHRONIC DISEASE

Writing towards the end of the eighteenth century, Hahnemann said that, having examined a large group of people, he could place the chronic diseases into three main classes. He christened them psoric, sycotic and syphilitic, of which the first was the largest group – say, seventy-five per cent – with the second and third about equally spread among his patients.

The psoric group is related to congestive states, skin troubles and deformities of spinal structure, and was also connected with tuberculosis. The sycotic types are related to gonorrhoeal complaints, warts, catarrh, and rheumatism. The syphilitic types are related to cardiac and neurological troubles.

Of course, this did not mean that Hahnemann suspected venereal disease in twenty-five per cent of his patients – only that in these smaller groups their complaints ran to a pattern which suggested to him that there was this miasm – perhaps three or four generations back – in their heredity. A miasm appears in the dictionary as a noxious odour rising from a swamp – Hahnemann used the word as a kind of stigma, for he was writing long before the days of the microscope and before bacteriology became an exact science.

ALTERING THE SOIL

Homoeopaths have said they can alter the soil on which disease grows. Two doctors, John and Elizabeth Paterson of Glasgow, spent twenty years making bowel cultures, from which study came bowel nosodes – a nosocomium was an old-fashioned name for hospital, from a Greek root meaning disease.

These two bacteriologists and practitioners made homoeopathic remedies from the bowel flora and always in their minds there was an interplay between the bacteriologistic and clinical approach to each case. Nosodes are named after the types of baccilli – Dysentery compound, Morgan, Gaertner, Proteous, etc., and are given as a kind of booster for the constitutional remedy.

This is complicated homoeopathic thinking and nosodes should not be prescribed by amateurs, for they have long-acting effects and should only be given at long intervals to complement the constitutional remedy, which is usually given in low potency.

Unfortunately, both the Patersons died before a detailed symptomatology of the bowel nosodes could be made readily available for young doctors interested in this field. Their papers are scattered through many journals but it is a fruitful study, and I refer to it here to show that homoeopathic philosophy has tried to link up with a modern discipline like bacteriology.

Dr Gibson Miller tried to make succinct generalization of non-surgical disease about fifty years ago. He divided disease into three groups:

A.   Acute – self limiting: recovery or death.
B.   Chronic – with one of the three miasms in the heredity.
C.   Due to: (1) unhealthy environment; (2) the abuse of drugs; (3) physical or mental strain.

Today most young doctors would consider this

quite unscientific, for they have been taught to classify disease by the end results as found in the post-mortem room, or by the gross pathological changes as found in the hospitals.

THE TOXINS

Dr Miller's idea in the difficult chronic cases, was that the miasms or toxins could be found: (1) as a single toxin; (2) as two or three toxins co-existing but separate; (3) as two or three toxins combined in the one person; (4) as any one of the third section in combination with the others.

It is this kind of thing which makes homoeopathy difficult when treating chronic cases. These people are so full of cortizone and its derivatives that they must be persuaded to stop such noxious drugs – sometimes we give them *Nux vomica* to clear the picture and then, if they come back, we have a chance to get our medicines to work.

The enquirer into homoeopathy, however, would be well advised to treat only acute cases of illness and leave the chronic work to experts. This may seem a curious thing to advise but in a life time of experience I have found acute cases of illness easier to treat. Only the other day a new case arrived out of the blue. She was a spry old lady of eighty-nine who was suffering from dizzy spells. Her first question was 'Could Homoeopathy do me any harm? Reassured on this point, she was given *Conium* 30 (poison hemlock) for her vertigo was worse when she went to bed in the afternoon or at night. She was a bit deaf and short-sighted, she had had her winter cough for thirty years, and she was shaky when excited.

Well, here was the four-legged stool – cough, vertigo, deaf, nearly blind and if she comes back in a month she should feel easier. This type of chronic case is an exception.

CHAPTER FIVE

TAKING THE CASE AND ASSESSING SYMPTOMS

Those readers who have had the curiosity to read this far will have realized that homoeopaths tackle a new case in quite a different manner from an allopathic doctor. To begin with, we have accepted Hahnemann's ideas which can be summarized as follows:

1. Disease is disharmony.
2. Like can be cured by like (*similia similibus curentur*).
3. Cure is the restoration of harmony.
4. Cure takes place from above downwards, then from within outwards.
5. The quantity of the drug required is in inverse ratio to the similarity of the symptoms.
6. If a drug in its crude state is poisonous to the Vital Force, it can be effective in attenuated dilutions.
7. Do not repeat a medicine if patient is improving.
8. Suppress nothing – pus, eczemas, temperatures, sweat.
9. Arndt-Schultz Law applies:
   Small stimuli – encourage life activity
   Medium stimuli – impede life activity
   Strong stimuli – stop or destroy life activity
10. The parts of a patient are not greater than the whole. (Consultants do not appreciate this.)

If a doctor can convince himself of the reasonableness of these ideas, and tries out a few of our well-proven remedies in his practice he will realize certain benefits:

1. The *safety* of homoeopathy – no side effects.

2. The *cheapness* of our medicines, as compared with allopathic ones.
3. The *gentleness* of our treatment – invaluable with the very old and the very young.
4. The *certainty* of improvement if we can hit on the exact *simillimum*.

The tyro, however, must strive to learn all he can about the drugs he is using, otherwise he cannot match them to the illness. It can be great fun – he gets a mental picture of the drug then fits it to his mental picture of the patient.

DR JOHNSON – THE SULPHUR TYPE

I have always been fond of the great Dr Samuel Johnson – even when I could not really afford it, I bought all the books I could find about that fascinating character, and still have most of them, though I sold the two-volume first edition dictionary to an American once, at a fine price, when hard up as a medical student.

In my opinion, Dr Johnson is the typical *Sulphur* type. All this from Boswell's Life of Johnson:

1. Standing is the worst position for a *Sulphur* patient. Old Sam when young paid his friends to carry him to school.
2. Patients requiring *Sulphur* have pronounced mental symptoms: they are melancholy minded, they worry about their soul's salvation. They are full of fears, hypochondriacal, peevish, bad-tempered, afraid of death. Sam was all those things.
3. *Sulphur* types are untidy, dirty, and glory in it. When Sam defended the sanity of his friend Christopher Smart he wrote:

   Another charge against him was that Smart

disliked clean linen. I have no passion for it myself.

4. Sam's person had an offensive odour. Sam once reproved a woman whispering to her friend: 'Madam, you are wrong! I do *not* smell, I may stink, but it is you who smell!'

5. *Sulphur* types love sweets and fat. At the Thrale's good table he soused his plum pudding with melted butter, and he put slices of buttered toast into his chocolate.

6. Patients requiring *Sulphur* are always thirsty. One day at Richard Cumberland's, when Sam asked for another cup of tea, Sir Joshua Reynolds reminded him that already he had drunk eleven cups. 'Sir' replied Sam. 'I do not count your glasses of wine, why should you number up my cups of tea?'

7. A *Sulphur* type feels full up after eating little. When Sam grumbled to his wife, Tetty, about her cooking, she said: 'Do not make a farce of thanking God for a dinner which, in a few minutes, you will protest as uneatable.'

8. His friend Sir Joshua Reynolds painted Sam many times with full red lips. The *Sulphur* types have thick, red negroid lips.

9. The *Sulphur* patient is usually deaf and short-sighted, as was Sam. He had catarrh of the middle ear and Sir Frederick Treves said his defective eyesight was the result of corneal leucomas, the product of tuberculous keratitis.

10. Sam had the typical *Sulphur* itch. Sir Russell Brain said that it was tuberculous in origin. Sam lived to be seventy-three and at the autopsy he was found to have emphysema, peritoneal inflammation, and ascites: with cystic changes in his kidneys.

He could have done with *Sulphur*, and perhaps the nosode *Psorinum*. I may have dwelt too long on Dr Samuel Johnson, but he will serve to impress on the mind of the learner of homoeopathy the perfect picture of a patient requiring *Sulphur*.

Such a one would come into the consulting room, brusque, dirty, untidy – the real ragged philosopher type – and would sit down before being asked. If you remarked politely that it was a fine day, he would reply that he had not come to discuss the weather. If the learner gets to know the type he is well on the way to knowing our great polychrest *Sulphur* – a homoeopathic remedy of great benefit to many, and in my experience often required by parsons.

THE MENTAL SYMPTOMS

Perhaps a little explanation is required of Hahnemann's fourth postulate – that cure takes place from above downwards, then from within outwards. This progression is not as marked today as in Hahnemann's time, but it still holds good as regards the mental symptoms – which the repertories go into in great detail and which homoeopaths regard as being of first importance (most disharmony starts in the mind).

For instance, Dr Johnson's appearance gave the first clue to *Sulphur* – but appearances are deceptive and much stronger clues are under 'Mind' in the repertories: anxiety, irritability, fear of imbecility, aversion to work, restlessness, religious mania – all give *Sulphur* in large type. Kent's repertory devotes ninety-five pages to mental symptoms.

The psychiatrist looks on the mental symptoms of his patient from quite a different angle. He may write down all the symptoms the patient gives – but he is looking for a diagnosis, not a matching drug. When he gets the symptoms he tries to interpret them according to his own ideas, or that of his mentors, Freud, Jung or Groddeck.

If, for example, a young woman comes to him complaining of morning sickness in the early months of pregnancy, he may tell her that her symptoms suggest she does not want her child, and that the sickness is her subconscious desire to get rid of it. The homoeopath takes her case with care, he knows he has a battery of remedies to choose from: she may require *Ipecachuana, Pulsatilla, Sepia, Nux vomica, Cocculus*, or a host of others, but he looks for his four-legged stool – four definite symptoms in the history on which he can build his choice. To quote Dr Ledermann: 'The homoeopathic physician is not concerned with the various theories of mental functioning, nor with the dynamics of the mind.' (*British Homoeopathic Journal*, October 1961.)

BRITAIN'S MOST POISONOUS PLANT

Another remedy which the beginner must know thoroughly is *Aconitum napellus* – known to herbalists as monk's hood or wolf's bane. It is a member of the botanical family *Ranunculaceae*, from which we have six well used homoeopathic drugs, including *Ranunculus* which is almost a specific against the after pains of shingles (a specific is a word homoeopaths seldom use). It is said to be Britain's most poisonous plant. Three milligrammes are sufficient to kill a horse, and Plutarch gives an account of Mark Antony's starving army grubbing up the roots with the result that 'every man died in paroxysm'. (D.M. Gibson, M.B., B.Sc., F.R.C.S., F.F.Hom., *British Homoeopathic Journal*, July 1964.)

The symptoms of acute poisoning by this plant are well recorded:

1. There is at once a burning in the mouth and throat and a tingling all through the body.
2. Thereupon cold sweats break out, with a feeling of deadly chill and numbness.
3. Intense pain is felt in the head, neck, back, and in the heart, and in about three hours death ensues from total circulatory failure.
4. A horrible death, from a feeling of awful terror.
5. Blindness, deafness and mental stagnation occur just before death.

I have gone into the graphic result of the crude alkaloid, for it helps the understanding of how the potentized version can be used for the good of mankind. I myself am fond of this remedy, for my mother kept a special store of *Aconitum* 6c for her own private use. She was red-faced, with a high blood-pressure, and was simply terrified of being laid up with a cold. It was during the First World War, she was committee-minded, and had to keep going, and she said to her two sons that *Aconitum* could stop her colds in twenty-four hours. She said it soothed her just to take one powder. During the awful influenza outbreak in 1918 she dished *Aconitum* out to all her friends and most of them survived, though 500 young Americans died on a troopship in the Clyde from this virulent strain of the illness.

Therefore, if I meet with a plethoric, full-blooded person who is coming down with a sudden chill and is full of an anxiety that is quite out of all proportion to the symptoms, I think of *Aconitum* at once.

Fear is the first clue, then *suddenness*, then *thirst*, then alternate feelings of *hot* and *cold*. All the pains are *severe* – especially headaches – and there may be *nose-bleeds* and *vertigo*. Eyes grow *dim* and there is often *earache*. If one gets four of these symptoms in an active, full-blooded person, one can be sure of helping them with *Aconitum*, in any potentized dose.

Dr Gutman remarks that the pains characteristic of *Aconitum* are 'unbearable', but that the drug has an affinity for the trigeminal nerve. (William Gutman, M.D., 'Aconitum Napellus', *British Homoeopathic Journal*, October 1959. I have used it in high potency in migraines and it has several successes to its credit – but, for the best results, it must be given to full-blooded, active patients, and not to the nervy, subdued woman. Dr Gutman also writes that the usual habitat of *Aconitum* is in the high mountain regions, where the plant is obviously able to resist the relative anoxia, so that the drug should be thought of in 'mountain sickness'. Incidentally, where a plant grows should be of interest to enquirers into homoeopathic drugs; for instance, *Arnica montana* – our remedy for bruises – grows on the mountainsides, and if a sheep slips off a ledge it knows by instinct to nibble a bit of *Arnica* if available.

RHEUMATISM

Two drugs widely used for rheumatism, with good results, are *Bryonia alba* and *Rhus toxicodendron*. Rheumatoid arthritis is one of the most interesting of the articular rheumatic diseases. Fifty years before Hahnemann published the *Organon*, Dr William Oliver – originator of the 'Bath Bun' – wrote: 'Tis certain, a most stubborn distemper, and has baffled all the professors of physick that ever appeared in the world. The cause lies too deep for any medicine or method yet known to come to the bottom of it.' (L.G.C. Martin, M.B., B.Sc., M.R.C.P., M.F.Hom., 'Rheumatism in History and Homoeopathy', *British Homoeopathic Journal*, July 1966.)

So it has been with us a long time. Mary, Queen of Scots suffered from it, as did Christopher Columbus, Renoir, and Sir Alfred Munnings.

My old professor of medicine, Professor Adam

Patrick, said in his introductory lecture on rheumatism, 'This is a disease of the middle class – a class to which I have the honour to belong. It rarely appears among the lower orders of society in Dundee, or among the well to do.' When I asked him for his explanation of this, he said he thought it was because most of the poor lived 'couthy' – comfortably – in single end flats, stone built, which were always warm. When they got on in the world and got council houses, they got rheumatism from changes in temperatures – they could not afford to heat their dwellings as formerly. Those clinical observations are valuable but often neglected.

White bryony is found in the hedgerows of Europe, and belongs to the botanical family of the *Cucurbitaceae*. It has long tendrils to help it climb the hedges. Most plants are dextral: they climb against the sun in the northern hemisphere, but two exceptions are the hop, which is sinistral, and bryony, which sends feelers up clockwise and anti-clockwise – thus giving it a strong stability. The patient requiring bryony is one whose aches and pains are worse for motion of any kind.

Gutman says that this type of patient is often to be found among the business community – he is cautious, methodical, easily irritable, when ill he just wants to be left alone, and he feels better for pressure – if the pains are in his right chest, that is the side on which he will lie in bed.

As old Dr E.B. Nash wrote years ago: 'It makes no difference what the name of the disease is, if the patient feels greatly better by lying still and suffers greatly on the slightest motion, and the more and the longer he moves the more he suffers, *Bryonia* is the first remedy to be thought of, and there must be very strong counter-indications along other lines that will rule it out.' (E.B. Nash, M.D., in his textbook *Leaders in Homoeopathic Therapeutics*.) Dr Hering also stresses this modality (modality is a clumsy word for the state or condition): 'Joints red, swelling, stiff, with stitching pain from slightest motion.'

Another key symptom is dryness of all mucous membranes which leads to excessive thirst; among the important mental symptoms are anxiety and a morose ill-humour.

Do not think of *Bryonia* only in connection with rheumatism. It does great work in pleurisy and is frequently needed in pneumonias. The sudden onset may have called for *Aconitum*, but *Bryonia* may follow with advantage, and it can be followed by *Rhus toxicodendron*, another of our stand-bys for rheumatism.

THE OPPOSITE MODALITY

Once the beginner has got the symptoms of *Bryonia* fixed in his mind, he should consider *Rhus toxicodendron* (poison ivy) which has the curious feature of the opposite modality – the pains the patient has are always better when moving about and most severe when at rest. It is a grand remedy for persons who suddenly get cold and stiff after being exposed to dampness.

Dr Roland Zissu of Paris has gone carefully into the action of *Rhus toxicodendron* on the anatomical elements in the body. (Dr Roland Zissu, Paris, 'The Action of Rhus Toxicodendron in Rheumatology', *British Homoeopathic Journal*, January 1967.)

He states that *Rhus toxicodendron* has definite action on:

the skin and nervous system (Ectoderm derivatives)

respiratory and digestive mucosa (Entoderm derivatives)

muscles and fibrous connective (Mesoderm derivatives)

tissue, tendons, ligaments and (Mesoderm derivatives)

cervical ganglions (Mesoderm derivatives)

Ectoderm is the outer layer of the primitive embryo.

Entoderm is the innermost layer of the primitive embryo.

Mesoderm is the middle layer of the primitive embryo.

These morphological terms are given to show how this remedy acts on the very core of being.

Dr Zissu states:

In fact, *Rhus tox*, is an important remedy in rheumatology. Major indications derived from its physiopathological actions explain in great part its patho-genetic signs. It can be valuable simillimum in all aspects of rheumatic disease, but more particularly in those which most frequently display its major characteristics and essential modalities; less in acute rheumatism than in sub-acute rheumatism; less in chronic progressive polyarthritis and in ankylosing spondylitis than in 'gouty rheumatism', less in the arthroses than in articular rheumatism; more in the large joints where musculo-tendinous and ligamentous elements are of importance, as much from the static as from the dynamic point of view; and lastly, in cellulitis, whether the cause be infectious or diathesic.

In daily practise *Rhus tox.* is often prescribed, for its pathogenetic signs are frequently found, but care should be taken not to be easily satisfied with a few key-notes. This, indeed, is the *raison d'être* for materia medicas and repertories, and it is not the purpose of this paper merely to repeat what they say. We would, however, make a few personal comments. The classic alternation of *Bryonia* and *Rhus tox.* is justified because their respective physiopathological actions are complementary. But experience has shown that these two remedies are more often effective given in succession than alternately. The prescription of *Bryonia* and *Rhus tox.* in alternation, though often justified in poly-articular lesions, where it has the approval of the materia medica, is often in practice followed by a prescription of one or the other in isolation. These two remedies frequently have as complementaries rheumatology *Arnica* or *Ruta*, but many others are equally valuable.

SCIENTIFIC RESEARCH

Rheumatism is perhaps the biggest cause of absenteeism and illness in Britain. Rheumatic clinics are springing up all over the country, with princely sums given for research. That research, however, is as usual directed to a classification of all the various types of rheumatism – at least twenty – and brave efforts are being made by the young researchers to find the cause of this crippling disease.

In my time as a student, the streptococcus was supposed to be the chief offender and tonsils were whipped out as a matter of routine if a child had 'growing pains'. Aspirin was the allopathic stand-by then, and it is now superseded by butazolidine, cortizone and its derivatives, and indocid, but the wise practitioner is becoming increasingly disenchanted with them, because of the serious side-effects. Lately, a consultant physician Dr Wyburn-Mason claims that rheumatoid arthritis is the result of protozoal infection – a minute one-cell animal said to cause malaria as well. He suggests treatment with the new drug, Clotrimazole.

If only the researchers could be persuaded to give a serious scientific trial to our well documented, safe, cheap, easily taken remedies, such as *Bryonia, Rhus tox., Cimicifuga, Causticum, Ruta,* and *Rhododendron,* they might be surprised. None is a specific for this protean illness, but if the symptoms are taken carefully and given time to act in favourable circumstances, surely the sufferers should be allowed the chance to try medicines which, if they do them no good, can certainly do them no harm.

Cimicifuga (black snake-root) is often used for spinal rheumatism, stiff necks and lumbagos. *Causticum* (potassium hydrate) has many symptoms of tearing pains and great weakness. *Ruta* (rue-bitterwort) is used for flexor tendon strains. *Rhododendron* (snow rose) is useful for swellings of small joints and for gout in the big toe.

HOMOEOPATHY AND PREGNANCY

I have said that acute work is easier than chronic work in homoeopathy because the patient's system is not clogged up with nostrums of all kinds. That is why we get good results working with children, and many grateful parents become lifelong homoeopathic patients because of some dramatic result with a child in the family.

About five years ago a young woman came to me to say her first child had been stillborn, and that she was now nearing her full time in her second pregnancy and dreading the event. She was perfectly healthy and was given a dozen powders of *Caulophyllum* 30 – blue cohosh, known as squaw root to the North American Indians. She produced a fine boy without trouble in a short labour, and, though she had a narrow pelvis, no forceps were required, to the astonishment of the midwife and her doctor. This lady appears to have many friends adding to the population in Fife, for they now demand the same powders. By using *Caulophyllum* I never once had to use forceps in my thirty-year practice.

Let us consider *Belladonna* (deadly nightshade) in potency. I think it was Sir John Weir who said: 'When one comes across a patient, hot as a hare, dry as a bone, red as beet, mad as a hen, blind as a bat – think at once of Belladonna!' Boericke's repertory lists the following symptoms: 'Skin – dry and hot, Face –

scarlet, Mouth – dry, Eyes – sensation as if half closed, Mind – patient lives in a world of his own. The first description is easier to remember ...'

TWO CASES

If the reader will forgive a personal recollection, I well remember my first day in practice, when I got a call to two patients in the same road in a prosperous suburb of Glasgow.

The first call was on a small girl of nine, the only child of very fussy parents. They lived in a large villa and had never been seen before. She had all the *Belladonna* symptoms – a good going scarlet fever – and I was comforted to hear that the local practitioner's girl next door was down with the same symptoms. Irene got *Belladonna* 30 – six powders – and next day her temperature had gone down from 104°F to 99°F – though I was called out again at night when it went up. I repeated the *Belladonna* in higher potency, and she never looked back. She was kept indoors for ten days, and she amused herself by phoning up her little pal next door every afternoon and comparing notes.

The doctor's daughter got the new sulphanilamides, and became very depressed. This was not helped by seeing Irene playing in her garden for three weeks while she remained in bed for a month. The doctor was uncharitable enough to maintain stoutly that Irene could not have had scarlet fever, until she was made to go in and show him her skin peeling on hands and feet.

The other case, further up the road, was not without its amusing side. It was the largest house in the district and there were two cars drawn up outside – both much more impressive than my second-hand Wolseley. The first belonged to the local doctor whose child was ill. His patient was the master of the house, an old boy of eighty. The second car belonged to a lady doctor, whose patients were the two unmarried daughters of the house.

Both doctors came out together while I was standing on the doorstep. They would have ignored me completely had not the maid, who was showing them out, said cheerfully: 'Ah – here's my doctor at last, now we will be getting somewhere. Come right in.'

Apparently the whole family was down with influenza, and the elderly Hebe simply had to get up to see to the household chores. She was a patient of my brother's – but lately gone off to the war. All she said was: 'I've got the 'flu again doctor – in fact, we've all got it! No need to examine me, your brother always gave me Gelsemium for it and it works like a charm. Just give me six powders, and I'll be able to stay on my feet and look after the other three, and will you drop these three prescriptions in at the chemists on your way home – and tell him to send them out today certain!'

I could not help glancing at the prescriptions – every one was different, the old boy was getting a mixture of tinct. opium camphoratae, tinct. ipecacuanhae and syrupi tolutani, and the old maids were getting aspirin and veganin.

This story helps to illustrate why homoeopaths are not popular with the ordinary doctors – it took about five years before the local man, whose daughter had had scarlet fever, would even nod to me in the street.

A curious fact about scarlet fever is that among my 2,000 patients, I saw about a dozen cases in 1940, about nine in 1941, and about six in 1942, and since then none for twenty years. I had almost forgotten what it looked like – the circum-oral pallor, the liquid eyes, the intense thirst – until a year or two before I retired, when I saw two cases. All did well on *Belladonna*, which is one drug whose symptoms match the disease almost perfectly, and which, to me at least, is adequate proof of the homoeopathic principle. It also dilates the pupils of the eyes and its active principal, atrophine, was once used by the ladies of Italy to glamourize their eyes.

Scarlet fever is caused by the streptococcus, and I have noticed that red-haired people take the disease more acutely than others.

CHILDREN'S AILMENTS

The best book on children's ailments treated by homoeopathy is *Children's Types* by the late Dr D.M. Borland, in which he tries to differentiate between the various groups – the fat ones requiring the anti-psoric *Calcarea carbonica* (carbonate of lime), the ones with swollen tonsils requiring *Baryta carb.* (carbonate of baryta), the nervy ones requiring *Arsenicum alb.*, and the weepy ones requiring *Pulsatilla*, and so forth.

Pulsatilla is the wind-flower and it is a grand remedy for measles, just as *Drosera* (sundew), that unusual insect-eating plant, in potentized form works wonders with whooping-cough. A good remedy for worms is *Cina* (worm seed) this works well in dogs as well as children). For Enuresis – bed wetting – many a mother saves her laundry bill by giving her child *Equisetum* (horse-tail, or scouring rush).

Asthma in children is another field where homoeopathy has proved successful. In my experience the psoric child often develops an infantile eczema after vaccination, and if this is suppressed it leads to a troublesome asthma which is very difficult to treat. We start with a tree remedy, *Thuja occidentalis* (arbor vitae), to get rid of the ill effects of the vaccination, then follow this with the nosode *Sycotic* co. This might be called altering the soil in which disease grows. Then we take the asthma symptoms as they appear, paying particular attention to periodicity.

The above is a kind of bird's eye view of how to go about children's complaints, and is by no means complete. But if I am proud of anything in more than thirty years of practice, it is that I have never lost a child under my care and the bulk of my children's work was done in the war years, when some got scant attention, with the fathers away and the mothers at munitions.

CHAPTER SIX

THE DEVELOPMENT OF HOMOEOPATHY

Dr Samuel Hahnemann was married twice. His first wife was a good Hausfrau, who presented him with eleven children, two boys and nine girls. One son died in infancy, the other married young and escaped the rigid tyranny of his upbringing by going abroad where he was never heard of again. This was an increasing sorrow to his father, who had been too busy fighting the establishment to have much to do with his children's upbringing.

Melanie, his second wife, was as pretty as her name. She was a fashionable French lady of uncertain origin, aged thirty-three when she married Hahnemann, who was then seventy-nine. It is said she wore trousers, had a mind of her own, and might be called a forerunner of Women's Lib. Before her marriage she persuaded the doctor to make a will leaving all his early capital to his daughters. However, after she had established the old man in the fashionable Paris society so familiar to her, she doubled his fees and cut him off entirely from his

daughters, who had no love for their young
stepmother.

Melanie gave the old man ten years of happiness,
and when he died she buried him beside two of her
former conquests. After fifty-five years, by the
generosity of wealthy American homoeopaths, both
were moved to Pere Lachaise Cemetery, the most
famous in France, containing the graves of Heloise
and Abelard, Moliere, Balzac, Rossini, and many of
France's immortals.

Melanie, before the old man died, adopted a
daughter, Sophie, whom she married to Karl von
Bönninghausen, the doctor son of one of
Hahnemann's most faithful followers. She took the
young couple into her home, and helped build up a
prosperous homoeopathic practice in spite of the fact
that Dr Carl Bönninghausen had tried repeatedly to
buy from Melanie all the written records of the
founder. A curious situation – Melanie helped the son,
while his father wanted the notes. But Melanie would
not part with them, even to Dr Dunham of America,
who could not raise the prohibitive price of 50,000
dollars she asked for them. Historians have called her
mean because of this.

Dr Curie, grandfather of Madame Curie of radium
fame, helped to establish homoeopathy in England.
He became interested in *Drosera*, (the plant sundew)
which had gained a reputation for helping
tuberculosis, especially laryngeal phthisis. He tried
three experiments on cats, who are not liable to that
disease, by feeding them with *Drosera*, and sure
enough, they took tuberculosis. This is one of the very
few experiments homoeopaths have ever done on
animals.

The father of Dame Ivy Compton-Burnett, the
distinguished novelist, was Dr James Compton-

Burnett, a leading homoeopathic physician in the last decade of the nineteenth century. He practised in Liverpool, Chester and London, and his friend and biographer was Dr J.H. Clarke whose three-volume *Dictionary of Materia Medica* is required reading for homoeopathic physicians. Dr Compton-Burnett was an aggressive type, and he tried his best to demonstrate how homoeopathy could alter the soil on which disease grows, especially cancer, where he had recorded successes in reducing tumours.

AMERICAN HOMOEOPATHY

Homoeopathy was received like a new religion in the United States and had many followers. Pride of place goes to Dr Constantine Hering, who wrote *Guiding Symptoms* in ten volumes in 1879, and tried out new drugs on himself. But perhaps the greatest American of them all was Dr James Tyler Kent. A great teacher – Sir John Weir was one of his students – Kent was a prolific writer and a fine prescriber. He was never tired of advocating the single dose of the single remedy, never to be repeated as long as improvement lasted. His monuments are his *Repertory of Homoeopathic Materia Medica* and his *Lectures on Homoeopathic Materia Medica*.

Another American was Dr E.B. Nash, whose *Leaders in Homoeopathic Therapeutics* is written in a lively style and is my favourite bedside reading. One has only to read his remarks on *Colchicum autumnale* (meadow saffron) to realize his humility. Allopaths think of *Colchicum* for gout but for homoeopaths it has many uses, and one of its modalities is that the smell of food cooking is anathema to the patient.

SUPPORT IN HIGH PLACES

In one respect homoeopathy has been lucky: it has

always had support from those in high places who favoured it with patronage. The first was Dr Harvey Quin, an exuberant Irishman born at the tail end of the eighteenth century, whose mother may have been the Duchess of Devonshire. He moved in exalted circles and had wit and charm, which brought him to the notice of society who were eager to try the new fashion in medicine. Quin was also a good prescriber and, as was mentioned earlier, did much to advance homoeopathy in England.

In 1923 Dr John Weir of Glasgow became Physician-in-Ordinary to the then Prince of Wales – later the Duke of Windsor. He continued in that appointment during the brief Reign of Edward VIII, and was then personal physician to Queen Maud of Norway from 1929 to her death in 1938, when he was made a Knight Grand Cross of the Royal Order of St Olav. In 1936 he became physician to Queen Mary, and remained her friend and physician until her death in 1953. In 1936 he was also appointed physician to the Duke and Duchess of York. When the Duke became King George VI, Sir John Weir was appointed Physician to the Royal Household, and continued to hold that office in the household of Queen Elizabeth II. He was created C.V.O. in 1926, K.C.V.O. in 1932 and G.C.V.O. in 1939, and in 1949 he received the Royal Victorian Chain. His main contribution to homoeopathic literature was *Forty Years of Homoeopathic Practice*.

The present holder of the Royal appointment is Dr Margery Blackie, Dean of the Faculty of Homoeopathy. She is the first of her sex to hold this high appointment.

Dr Blackie has done heroic work in the Royal London Homoeopathic Hospital by organizing tutorials for qualified practitioners, and the courses are becoming increasingly popular year by year. Tutorials in the winter are also held in the Glasgow Homoeopathic Hospital under the able guidance of the superintendant, Dr Hamish Boyd, son of the late Dr W.E. Boyd.

HOMOEOPATHIC LITERATURE

In a short book of this type it is not possible to mention all those who have contributed towards the development of homoeopathy. One of the first, however, was Dr Richard Hughes, whose *Manual of Pharmaco-Dynamics* was one of the best of early textbooks. Dr Hughes was an advocate for low potencies prescribed on pathological signs rather than on symptoms. Each year the Faculty arrange a memorial lecture in his memory.

Mention should also be made of another distinguished lady, Dr Margaret L. Tyler, daughter of Sir Henry Tyler, who gave a large sum towards the foundation of the London Hospital in the mid-eighties. Dr Tyler, a gifted writer, worked closely with Sir John Weir, and wrote *Homoeopathic Drug Pictures*, a volume which is as fresh today as when it was written.

Since her time the standard of homoeopathic literature has steadily improved, perhaps by her example. Dr Charles Wheeler also had the gift of writing, and his *Principles of Homoeopathy* is a classic of its kind. Dr D.N. Gibson, now retired to Canada, has for many years written the most delightful articles in the magazine *Homoeopathy* on the various drugs popular to homoeopaths, in which he gives their origins and their places in the botanical families.

More recently two other books have been published, one by Dr G. Ruthven Mitchell entitled *Homoeopathy* and the other by Dr Margery Blackie with the title of *The Patient, Not the Cure*.

HOMOEOPATHIC SUPPLIERS

Homoeopathic medicines were at one time made up by practitioners who had the leisure and ability to do so. Indeed, some became so confident in the potency of their drugs that they thought a sniff of the right medicine was all that was was required. Today, though, they can be bought, and for the supply of medicines and homoeopathic accessories, I have always dealt with A. Nelson & Co., 73 Duke Street, London, but there are others equally reliable, such as: Ainsworth's Pharmacy, 38 New Cavendish Street, London W1; E. Gould & Sons, 14 Crowndale Road, London NW1; Kilburn Chemists Ltd., 216 Belsize Road, London, NW6; The Galen Pharmacy, 1 South Terrace, South Street, Dorchester; Freemans, 7 Eaglesham Road, Clarkston, Glasgow. All of these could no doubt supply handy packs of the drugs mentioned in this book.

CHAPTER SEVEN

USEFUL INFORMATION

If a young graduate is interested in homoeopathy, he should get in touch with the Royal London Homoeopathic Hospital, Great Ormond Street, London, WC1N 3HR, and ask to be put in touch with the Secretary of the Faculty of Homoeopathy, the professional body for homoeopathic doctors.

The Faculty, incorporated by Act of Parliament in 1950, is responsible for the standards of postgraduate training required by qualified practitioners. It runs winter tutorials and sets examinations for associates and members.

It is possible to get homoeopathic treatment under the National Health Service and anyone wishing to

learn more about the subject should write to the
Secretary-General, The British Homoeopathic
Association, 27A Devonshire Street, London, W1N
1RJ. This registered charity is over sixty years old,
and is composed of people from all walks of life. It
publishes its own journal, *Homoeopathy*, and is most
helpful in putting would-be patients in touch with their
nearest homoeopathic doctor. For a small annual
subscription, the members of the Association are kept
in touch with homoeopathic thought.

A medical student who has the curiosity to read this
book may ask with justification: 'Why has
homoeopathy, with all the good points outlined in this
book – safety, certainty, cheapness, gentleness – not
swept the country and become an integrated part of
medical care?' The short answer is Mass Medication –
dramatic discoveries such as antibiotics and
cortizone, no encouragement from the establishment
or the academics, and bureaucratic control.

Another point is that the young doctor inside the
National Health Service is assured of a good income
with ancillary benefits and an adequate pension at
sixty-five. He does not have to build up a practice, or
to go for tutorials at his own expense. His young wife
will tell him to put security first. But he need never
fear that homoeopathy will die out as a system of
medical therapeutics, for up and down the country
there are little groups of people waiting for
homoeopathic doctors to take the place of those who
have gone before.

In Russia, homoeopathy persists and flourishes as
never before, proving that the juggernaut of state
control can never crush the individual, no matter how
heavily bureaucracy comes down on personal freedom.
In India alone, there are registered over 70,000
homoeopaths with state councils of homoeopathic

medicine in Calcutta and Trivendrum, and many directors and registrars in various states throughout India. Homoeopathy flourishes in France, Germany, Mexico, Argentina and Brazil. In the United States, the once prosperous homoeopathic societies are being revived due to dissatisfaction with the enormous cost of present-day medicine. In that country, practitioners have to take out enormous insurance premiums in case they are sued by dissatisfied patients. The malpractice insurance rates run from 808 dollars for a general practitioner to 12,650 dollars for a neuro-surgeon – no wonder physicians in California and New York have been on strike.

One of the pleasant things about homoeopathic practice is that, as a rule, one is dealing with people of intelligence and by the system of individual treatment, one gets to know them as friends. I myself have never heard of a homoeopathic patient who wanted to sue the doctor – perhaps because they all realize that the doctor has done his best for each individual under his care, and has done him good.

That is why we can say with Shakespeare: 'We few, we happy few, we band of brothers.' But if we want to become more than a happy few, we must be more assertive in putting forward the claims of homoeopathy, and those who have benefited from the treatment must tell their friends.

A doctor already established but dissatisfied with the results and trends in modern medicine can quite easily start with a few of the more familiar remedies suggested in this book and try them out on his patients for himself.

He will get all the co-operation possible from:

The Royal London Homoeopathic Hospital,
Great Ormond Street, London, WC1N 3HR

Glasgow Homoeopathic Hospital,
1000 Great Western Road, Glasgow G12 0NR

Glasgow Homoeopathic Out-Patients Department,
5 Lynedoch Crescent, Glasgow, G3

Bristol Homoeopathic Hospital,
Cotham, Bristol, BS6 6JU

Tunbridge Wells Homoeopathic Hospital,
Church Road, Tunbridge Wells, Kent.

They are all in the National Health Service.